Testimonials

What People Are Saying

"*The Book of Joy* is a message that the world badly needs right now. The stories that the author shares leave the reader smiling at how beautifully whimsical moments are captured, giving us a powerful reminder to focus on the small joys that grace our every day when we remember to pay attention." - Elin Barton, a Coach, Entrepreneurial Community Builder and Author of *Ready, Set, Grit: Three Steps to Success in Life, Business and Pursuit of Happiness,* elinbarton.com

"Laura's words will wrap you up in a cozy blanket of warm light. She doesn't avoid the perils of modern life but brings her loving sense of peace and helps us understand how to transmute them into gold. It's relaxing and inspiring, all at the same time." - Amanda Fuel, Speaker's coach, NextLevelFuel.com

What People Are Saying

"Smiling, as I felt the essence of this book, I am reminded that life is an opening to new awareness and the power within us to embrace each day with fresh perspectives. A must-read for people who seek inner peace."- Teresa A. Huggins, Inspirational Speaker, Best-Selling Author, www.teresadhuggins.com

"Read this book like butterflies, read flowers, read it like poetry. Rest with one paragraph at a time and find the sweetness of joy there." – Halina Goldstein, Author, and Founder of the Joy Keepers Network, HalinaGold.com, www.joykeepers.org

"Taking the time to reflect on life's simple, pleasurable moments and memories can change one's heart and attitude, giving way to joy. A very inspirational read, especially for those of us who are lost in busyness." - Marianne Angelillo, Motivational Speaker, and Author of *Sharing My Stones*, matthewangelillo.com

The Book of Joy
Overcoming Life's Challenges

Laura (signature)

Laura Ponticello

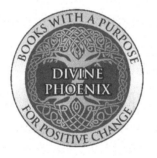

Divine Phoenix LLC
Auburn, New York

ISBN 978-0-9853915-7-7
1. Happiness
2. Self-Development

Book cover design by Christopher Moebs
Author photo © Laure Lillie Photography
Specific stock imagery © Dreamstime
Book cover Image: Photo 203954925
Morpho Butterfly Sunset © Oleksii
Kriachko
Dreamstime.com
Quotes: www.goodreads.com,
www.brainquote.com,
physchologytoday.com,
www.wikipedia.com
Illustration: Dreamstime.com © Svitlana
Baklytska

Printed in the United States of America

This book is the author's perception. No
medical advice is offered. All viewpoints
presented merely represent the author's
interpretation of events and experiences.

Dedication

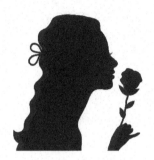

To Nana Rose, who taught me numerous life lessons. She imparted the wisdom to "Take time to stop and smell the roses in life."

"Find out where joy resides and give it a voice far beyond singing. For to miss the joy is to miss it all."

– Robert Louis Stevenson

Contents

The Significance of the Butterfly on the Front Cover and in Life

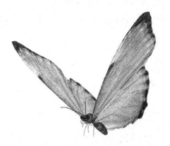

"Just when the caterpillar thought the world was over, it became a butterfly."

– English proverb.

I have always loved winged creators, especially butterflies. Ever since I was a young girl, I would chase them in the wind. Then, hoping to get as close as possible to their beauty, I offered a hug as a sign of affection.

Yet, it wasn't until years later that I learned that I needed to be quiet to present the butterfly a chance to rest on my shoulders.

In these moments, I turned off the exterior noise of the world around me, and I tuned into the whispers of my heart. As a result, I became one with nature.

So, I noticed a changing form of an oak tree in the distance. Its leaves are shifting color from green to yellow and also amber. A sign that nature is transforming itself into something anew.

A paradoxical mirror reflection exists today. For many times the grass beneath my feet felt barren as the storms of life erupted. But a knowing existed that Mother Earth was storing up nutrients during the dormancy period. Therefore, all that nature needs to sustain its growth is always available.

We, too, are constantly evolving like the transitioning oak tree and the butterfly emerging from the cocoon. Plus, shedding any residual layers that we don't need any more to become the most iridescent form of ourselves.

"We delight in the beauty of the butterfly but rarely admit the changes it has gone through to achieve that beauty." - Maya Angelou.

Preface

"What I am looking for is not out there; it is in me." – Hellen Keller

I invite you on a journey towards a blissful life. Together we will discover what makes you smile, what entices you to feel contentment, and how to infuse more joy into your daily life.

At the onset of a day, you decide how best to approach being alive. You can experience life from a perception of hopefulness, savoring the sheer fact that you have a gift ready to unfold in the present moment.

There are numerous invitations to achieve happiness in a single day.

Therefore, let's uncover what aspects of life excite you—peeling back the layers within you that store your deepest desires—creating room for happiness to become a reality.

However, first, you must relinquish the old to make room for the brand new. This process will require you to push past the comfort zone, step over fear to extract self-doubt, and allow for the energy flow of joy.

Once in alignment, you can live from a place of blissfulness.

For when you are joyful, you shine as a beacon of light. And you disperse light amidst the darkness. Thereby spreading seeds of love wherever you traverse.

With excitement for what is about to transpire as we explore what lies ahead for you,

Launa

"Happiness isn't what you find at the end of the road. It's right here. Right now." – Unknown

How Best to Interact with *The Book of Joy*

Bite-size nuggets tend to be easily digestible. So, you will find shorter chapters, bursts of real-life stories, and quotes that foster contemplation.

A conversational writing style permits you to sip the content as if we are sitting together like good friends enjoying a soothing cup of calming tea or a special latte filled with love.

The size of this book encourages you to carry it with you, open at any page, and refer back when you need a bit of refreshment.

Furthermore, you will discover *Points to Ponder* and *Reader Reflections,* which present an opportunity for you to pause and be contemplative.

Please take your time since this is not a race to the finish line. Read at your own pace. Absorb what feels right for you. Most importantly, find delight in the journey.

"The only question in life is whether or not you are going to answer a hearty 'YES!" to your adventure."

– Joseph Campbell

Introduction

Why Joy Now?

"Don't miss all the beautiful colors of the rainbow looking for the pot of gold."

– Anonymous

Due to the business of life, we have forgotten a powerful truth – that **joy is our natural state.**

Therefore, a personal call exists to experience life from a perspective of *joy*.

Studies show that taking time to appreciate pleasurable occurrences can make you happier.

"After all, it's the little moments that make up your life," according to Harvard Medical School, shares Kelly Bilodeau, Executive Editor Harvard Women's Health Watch.

Countless happenings transpire every day, presenting a chance to inhale life's fragrance. But if you neglect taking time to be present in the Now, you miss precious moments waiting to unfold like fresh flowering blossoms.

Maybe it's when you slow down to witness the beauty around you that ignites joy.

"Perfect happiness is a beautiful sunset, the grandchild's giggle, the first snowfall. It's the little things that make happy moments, not the grand events. Joy comes in sips, not gulps." – Sharon Draper

Joy is beckoning at the doorstep; however, you must be willing to permit its presence.

As you make room for joy, you become mindful of what makes your heart sing. And the stuff you once sweated in the daily routine of life now feels irrelevant.

Soon life becomes an enchanted walkway. You uncover steppingstones on the path of self-discovery and awaken to the insight that life can be joyful.

So, you leap ahead with happiness and approach life with excitement. Then you find magical occurrences are awaiting your arrival.

Chapter One

Making Space for Joy

"Anything I cannot transform into something marvelous, I let go."

– Anais Nin

My sister always kicked her clothes under the bed in our childhood. But, on the other hand, I liked to keep everything in pristine order.

My books were in symmetry on a bookcase. Jordache jeans lined up perfectly in my dresser drawer. And Converse® sneakers were polished as if not to showcase a speckle of dirt.

Additionally, a vanity table held my hairbrush and a purple grape crush lip balm. And I stored a journal with a key in the bedroom closet. Secret wishes were locked away, hoping that my dreams would manifest into reality one day.

Weird as it may sound, I found great pleasure in making my bed and tidying up my room. But my sister had a contradictory definition of an orderly room.

Despite multiple attempts to arrange her stuff neatly, she always relapsed to placing her clothes beneath the bed. Plus, she never really focused on keeping her room organized.

Because I was the elder, Mom always told me to set an example.

One day, Christina asked me, "Why do you bother nagging me? I know where everything is located in my room. I like it the way it is."

When the lightbulb hit me, one person's messiness might be their genuine sense of perfection.

Each of us interprets living areas entirely differently.

The concept of making space for joy varies and is subject to how you view life.

A friend recently told me, "Joy is like olive oil. It pours out quickly to flavor the vegetables of your life, or you have to shake the bottle in hopes that the last drop falls on the plate."

For me, joy is a feeling that cumulates from within. When I sit with a cup of tea in hand and start the day by writing in a journal, I find contentment.

Natural treasures that abundantly surround me in nature, such as a hummingbird fluttering on a hibiscus plant in the yard or the bunny rabbit hopping across the grass, yield a smile.

Witnessing flowers in the garden bloom as they move in the sun's direction creates cheerfulness.

Laughter with neighbor's children as we construct fairy gardens in the yard reminds me of childlike fun.

Special times with family create joyful occasions, especially when we gather to eat chicken barbeque on the 4th of July, followed by Mom's white cake with *Cool Whip* frosting.

We play Badminton as a family. Dad makes homemade strawberry ice cream with seasonal strawberries, crème, and rock salt that he churns in a giant ice cream bucket machine. And we eat every morsel.

Now, unique occurrences with my adult sister make me euphoric. We pour chilled Prosecco wine, drop frozen blackberries in the wine glasses, and laugh about childhood memories.

As you recall joy-filled moments, how do you define joy?

Point to Ponder: If I offered you a cup labeled "Joy," what would you place inside your cup of joy?

Take a few minutes to think about these questions.

For Reflection: "Realize deeply that the present moment is all you ever have. Make the NOW the primary focus of your life." - Eckhart Tolle

Chapter Two

Shifting to the Now

"Be happy in the moment, that's enough. Each moment is all we need, not more."
– Mother Teresa

Since we experience many human emotions, our joy litmus stick can change on any given day. One day you might feel elated. Another day, struggle even to find a speck of happiness.

Because life isn't an ideal sandwich with delicious fresh preserves and crème cheese, all of the time, you have to store up bits of JOY. Then you can lean into a reserve of JOY when you need it the most.

As you realize that life bestows a gift today, you forgo worrying about tomorrow.

And you can't change yesterday.

Instead, you can be present in the **Now.**

"In order to do the things, we love, the things we really love, we need to be present. When we are present in these activities, we get to experience them more deeply and experience the joy they bring to our lives." – Jack Heinbigner, author of *How Being Present Will Bring Joy to Your Life*.

Why does being present help create Joy?

First, you have time to reflect. It is necessary to allocate time for self-discovery. When you connect with yourself, thoughts and feelings arise surrounding what makes you happy.

In addition, you become mindful of the blessings in your life.

Instead of regretting what you don't have, you appreciate all the little things that add to the significant aspects of your life.

Reflective Exercise - Let's explore shifting attention to the present time.

First, begin by taking a deep breath.

Inhale to the count of three, exhale slowly. Repeat this pattern three times.

Sit still for a few minutes to quiet the mind. Feel your shoulders relax.

Let any distracting thought float away like puffy white clouds.

Release any worry into the Universe, as if they are being carried away by beautiful birds.

Place your hands on your heart.

Breathe into your heart.

Then begin to recite, "I am worthy of Joy. I am an open vessel to receive joy. I now claim my worthiness to be joyful and welcome joy into my life. My cup of life is overflowing with joy."

Inspired Idea: A good reminder is to utilize the breath as a gateway to becoming present in the Now. When you breathe, you awaken, ignite the senses, and attune your energy into a state of balance.

For Reflection: "Sometimes you need to sit quietly lonely on the floor in a quiet room to hear your own voice and not let it drown in the noise of others." - Charlotte Erikson.

Chapter Three

Claiming Room for You

"Make room for what matters... let go of what doesn't. It is that simple." – Livehappy.com

As you begin to expand the space for joy's arrival, you realize that claiming time for YOU is essential.

Due to life's busyness, we often negate a crucial vessel, ourselves.

How can you steer a ship without taking the helm? Even if the ship's course is predetermined, navigation is necessary.

To keep the ship on course, you need clarity of mind to direct it. If your energy is going in too many directions, you lose perspective. But if you are balanced, decision-making flows effortlessly, and you guide the ship safely into port.

The counterbalance is weaving all over the map. This tends to happen when we are out of balance.

There have been multiple occurrences when I was entirely off course. I forgot to take time to sit still and breathe into life. In addition, work was piling up with deadlines to meet and family commitments.

There wasn't a flashing light saying: "Get yourself back in balance."

Therefore, I have to remember to "Slow the pace."

If I leap out of bed engaging in the technological world first thing, I forgo allocating time to center myself.

Instead, I choose to stretch into life. This concept means allocating fifteen minutes at the onset of the morning to wake up, stretch the body, twinkle the toes, and drink a glass of water to hydrate.

As the day progresses, I find another chance to recalibrate. My cellular phone reminds me to allocate another stretch break at 3 pm to get the blood flowing and creative juices pumping.

Inspired Action: Mark on your calendar *Me Meeting Time.* No matter what, take this meeting with yourself. It will be the most important meeting of your life

Becoming Mindful for Joy

As I became aware of the desire to experience more joy, I realized that time is a precious gift. So, I decided to keep a sixty-four-hour time log. This process was necessary because I longed for additional time to experience aspects of life that I loved, such as walks with Bunny the dog, writing, and gardening.

I called this experiment "Becoming Mindful for Joy."

During a sixty-four-hour period, I logged my actions in three categories: Joyful, Necessary (buying groceries, paying bills, getting gas, cleaning house), or Delete (meaning I could let the action go).

If I felt uplifted or content, I labeled the action as Joyful. For a necessary task, I challenged myself to make the action FUN! For example, I now play dance music when vacuuming the house. My neighbor told me she listens to audiobooks for a more joyful experience when mowing the yard.

Point to Ponder: How can you infuse fun into necessary chores?

Time Matters - Before you commit to attending an event, or lunch request, ask yourself, "Do I want to spend my time performing this action? Will this act create joy? Is there a more efficient way to participate?"

Ask Yourself: What do you need to say no to say YES to Yourself?

Inspired Action: Review activities over the following few days to become mindful of what actions feel joyful and which actions you can release into the Universe.

For Reflection: "When you discover something that nourishes your soul and brings joy, care enough about yourself to make room for it in your life." – Jean Shinoda Bolen

Chapter Four

Clear The Clutter

"Clear clutter, make space for you."

– Magdalena Vandenberg

It is incredible how many personal belongings we collect over a lifetime.

Take a few minutes to walk around your house or apartment or scan your office, simply noticing your stuff. While some possessions you may love, other items collect dust and take too much space.

Certain household pieces can be sentimental and not the easiest to surrender. However, memories are stored in the heart, not necessarily in things.

For me, letting go wasn't easy. I was gifted numerous beautiful objects with emotional ties. Therefore, I started to take inventory, one room at a time. As I cleared the clutter, I held each item, asking, "Do I love it? Does the item bring me joy? Should I shift its location, or is it meant for another?"

21

What surprised me was freeing up space; I made room for *new energy to flow.*

The concept of letting go extends way beyond material possessions. Possibly it means reviewing relationships, how you allocate time, and, to be blunt, what you need to release because you have held on for far too long.

A letting go process led me to many beautiful intersections.

One lady (Kathy) said she looked for the Waverly chair fabric that matched her kitchen curtains for ten years.

Rebecca shared that her grandmother gifted her a piece of China with a rose pattern. However, during a recent family gathering, the item broke by accident. Given that I relinquished, the exact China pattern meant that she would now have a beloved collection intact.

Yet Fran is someone who I will never forget. She drove a black sports utility vehicle with dark windows and super shiny silver tire rims. And she had a huge personality.

Fran jumped out of her SUV, wearing Prada® sunglasses, a black jumpsuit with black flats, and holding her precious dog, Maxim.

She told me that her beloved Maxim has traveled with her ever since she adopted him. For a Pomeranian, he is soft to the touch. You couldn't miss him because a rhinestone collar clung to his neck, engraved with his name.

I held Maxim when Fran opened the trunk of her car. Then she asked me, "Do you have her? I literally can't wait to meet her."

"Yes," I reply. Yesterday, I had loaded her up and strapped her to the front seat of my car to make sure she was secure for the drive.

Like a scene out of the show, *The Sopranos*, I felt like we were getting ready to bury a body or do a massive hit.

Fran grabbed a sapphire blue blanket in the trunk of her car, shouting out, "I want her to be comfortable on the ride home."

By this point, the heat is getting to me.

23

Recently hormones have been all the place due to metabolic changes.

Yet Fran is as cool as a cucumber.

"Should I call her Helen? Does she seem like a Helen?" Fran inquires with calm composure.

Before I can utter a word, "Helen was my neighbor. She just died. I know she would want me to be happy."

She affirms, "Definitely a Helen."

"Helen always loved fairies. So, she will go to my sunroom, facing Helen's house. When the sun comes into my porch, her bronze wings will sparkle. I will know Helen is near me."

Fran began to place her (which she had just named Helen) in the blanket. Next, she closed the car door after placing Helen in the front passenger seat.

"Would you like to kiss Maxim goodbye?" asked Fran. I politely declined.

While driving off, she rolls down the car window, waves, and yells, "I just love my Helen."

After meeting Fran, I decided to head towards a garden center on the other side of town.

Here, I purchased a bird feeder with the money from the garden fairy.

When I returned home, I hung the feeder on the oak tree and reflected that "One person's lost treasure is another individual's pot of gold."

Points to Ponder: What are you holding on to, whether materialist or sentimental stuff that might serve another? What would you like to make room for in your life?

Chapter Fiᵛ

Evolving Be

"The only way to make sense ouᵗ ᵒᶠ change is to plunge into it, move with it, and join the dance." – Alan Watts

As we evolve, so does our way of thinking. We often find that the ideology learned in our younger years may no longer feel relevant. As a result, some previous ideas don't resonate, while other perceptions still seem relevant. So, we release outdated views, adapt beliefs, and explore original ways of thinking.

For me, a mindset of "Work hard to get ahead and make a difference in the world" is the sentiment of the times.

Working hard is inbred in me. I learned this belief from Dad. He taught me to "Never feel sorry for myself. Instead, put one foot in front of the other and move forward. Do something in life, contribute to society."

Yet when I reflect, I realize how much sports influenced me. Coach Bill was my friend's father and soccer coach. He exuded optimism and praised us for acting as a team. As a result, I learned to play fair even though we performed a competitive sport.

The coach encouraged us to project positivity. I would visualize a positive outcome, whether in school or work. Most of the time, the action came to be. Besides the power of visualization, I felt the act as if it had already transpired.

Performance athletes engage in this mindset. For example, I remember reading an article about tennis star Serena Williams sharing that the art of visualization was a game-changer.

"You need to see things happening and envision yourself in a fantasy world – and believe in that world – until it comes true," she said.

As time passed, I learned that I could not always control outcomes. This lesson wasn't easy for me.

Because sometimes, **the Universe has a bigger plan for you than you understand at the time.**

I didn't foresee curveballs, such as life occurrences that arrive without proper notice.

Due to the ideology of the times, I believed that marriage was a bound contract. Therefore, you stay married for sickness and in good health, bad or happy, no matter what. My Italian Catholic family emphasized "Remaining committed to the family before anything else," even if that meant self-sacrifice.

Let's face it - when you fall in love, you think love will be forever. Until the day that the magical gingerbread house comes crumbling down. Then you are left to reconstruct the broken pieces. Only to find that they don't fit back together at all.

During the divorce, I asked myself, "Why?"

I second-guessed myself. As I clung to the past, I felt stuck.

The more resistance to change, the deeper I experienced the pain.

Finally, after many restless nights, a thought emerged, "What if a gift exists in this circumstance?"

What if innovative opportunities in life are awaiting my arrival? What if...

I did not expect these thoughts. So, I began to explore further in a journal the above questions.

Point to Ponder: If each occurrence suggests a blessing, could there be a gift waiting for you?

As you realize what makes you joyful, old beliefs may surface.

A dear healer friend Bonita said, "Why are you replaying old-outdated tapes? If you do not like the recording of your life, change it!"

Playing old, outdated tapes never helps.

For Reflection: "It is not what you say out of your mouth that determines your life. It's what you whisper to yourself that has the most power." – HavingTime.com

Chapter Six

Suzie Sunshine

"Let us dance in the sun, wearing wildflowers in our hair..." - Susan Polis Schutz

My family likes to call me Suzie Sunshine because I tend to perceive the bright side of things. I am not the type who views the glass as half empty. On the contrary, I sense and feel the glass is overflowing.

In my human resource career, I had the most amazing personal assistant. She had excellent organizational skills and always kept me on schedule. Plus, she had something positive to say about her environment, hence a perfect match for me.

When she went out on family medical leave, I was assigned temporary help. Marla, the interim assistant, was never happy. She was wronged by her man, as she told me, and believed that everyone was out to get her.

I felt on edge each time Marla was near me. Yet, I attempted to redirect her towards positivity, given my utopic outlook. "Did you happen to notice the flowering cactus plant in the lobby? How about trying those delicious cookies that Jane brought in for the staff?" I would ask.

However, the more I focused on making Marla happy, the more I felt utterly drained.

I couldn't wait for my assistant to return from temporary leave! And I practically kissed the ground she walked on when she returned to work.

In hindsight, I now understand that Marla (the temp) must have been in much pain, given her negativity. Yet, I didn't need to respond to her behavior.

For Reflection, "Do not let the behavior of others destroy your inner peace." – His Holiness, Dalai Lama

My sister says, "You are like a magnet to attract individuals." For whatever reason, people gravitate towards me, always sharing their life stories. So, today is not an exception.

Bob and I intersect at the local bakery in town. He is six feet tall with peppercorn black and silver hair.

Immediately Bob begins to complain about the long line is at the bakery. "Who has time to wait? It is ridiculous that a sandwich takes this much time to prepare."

I respond with, "They are busy."

Bob yells across the counter, "Hey, what is taking so long?"

The gal behind the counter reacts, "We are super busy due to food orders. Take a chill pill!"

Bob rolls his eyes, telling me, "I have to get to an important meeting. I don't have time for this delay."

I inquire, "What type of sandwich did you order?"

"Egg salad on rye."

"Oh, I love their egg salad with the little olives?"

"Yes," he proclaims.

With a smile on my face, I react with, "Since you are impatient, why don't you leave? I will take your sandwich."

Bob doesn't appreciate my response.

Mom always says, "Treat another how you want to be treated." Yet, many times, that rarely happens.

Even on a perfect day, you encounter people like Bob.

The key is not to **let others rain on your parade.** People's actions can't steal your peace unless you permit them.

I bring up the story of Bob since **You can place anything you want in the cup of life that makes you happy.**

In parting ways, Bob inquires, "What do you do anyway?"

Before I can react, the lady with the red hat in line states, "Didn't you write a book recently?"

Months later, I crossed paths with Bob again at the local bakery. However, this time Bob looks different. Instead of a conservative business suit, he is wearing khaki pants with a light blue polo shirt. Also, his shoulders appear relaxed.

Bob imparts, "Responsibilities sucked the life out of me. I used to love reading *The New Times*. Plus, drinking a cup of strong coffee in the morning before my wife and kids woke up. I ran four times a week."

He continues, "I do not know what happened to me. Life became work. I am in the financial services business. Anyways, I am working on getting back to the man I used to be."

I respond, "You can never go back, only forward."

Afterward, we picked up our egg and olive sandwiches and bid goodbye.

Before walking out the door, Bob offers, "I acquired your book. It's been sitting on my desk. Then I stuck it in a drawer. Maybe this time, I will read it."

Inspired Action - The Five-Minute Positivity Pause

"Sometimes the most important thing in a whole day is the rest we take between two breaths."– Etty Hillesum

Allocating five minutes to rebalance is extremely helpful, especially when a stressful situation occurs.

If possible, remove yourself from the environment, and seek refuge even in the bathroom. You may be surprised how five minutes in a bathroom can help you regain composition. For example, before returning to a business meeting, I've sat on many toilets breathing to induce calmness.

In the article, *Five Reasons to Take a Breathe Before Responding*, we learn, "Taking a breath induces oxygen into your body and brain, which will help you stay calm and improve your thinking process."

Therefore, take a deep breath. Exhale slowly. As you breathe, know that you are calm.

Repeat and affirm, "I am calm. I encircle myself with the light of positivity. I am peaceful."

Feel the light of positivity flowing into you like rays of sunshine.

Then zip up yourself in the positive vibes, as if you are putting on a jacket of love.

Now you are ready to return to the situation with grace and calmness.

A good reminder – While you can't control the actions of others, you can choose your response. Often, the best course of action is no response until you are in a state of calmness.

If you can't remove yourself from the environment, you can envision a ring of golden light encircled with positivity surrounding you and the environment. And you can transmute fear into hope, and stress into peace, As well as, set the intention for the highest and best good for all involved in the current situation.

For Reflection: "In the midst of movement and chaos, keep stillness inside of you." – Deepak Chopra

Chapter Seven

Wishing on a Rainbow

"The way I see it, if you want the rainbow, you gotta put up with the rain."
– Dolly Parton.

By this time, the divorce is moving ahead. So, uncertainty exists for me, especially in my surroundings.

Furthermore, I have to acquire my parents a place to live. Currently, Dad lives at the guest house adjacent to my homestead because he works locally. Mom resides out of town due to caretaking for her aging father.

But today, Mom checks herself into a local retreat center in Skaneateles, New York, run by the Sisters of St. Francis.

My Aunt Joan accompanies Mom.

They say, "A rite of passage" exists for Mom, given her recent retirement and Papa's death.

Mom declares, "Aunt Joan and I will start a novena prayer to Blessed Mother Mary to help you attain a suitable home."

Linda, my real estate agent, calls me as Mom and Aunt Joan amp up the prayers.

Linda states, "I have a house to show you. I think you are going to like the house."

Meantime, Mom rings me, "A bat keeps awakening me at night, hitting the room's door. Constant banter on my door."

Mom is deathly afraid of bats. So now Mom's prayers include the safe passageway of the bats to another locale.

I agree to meet Linda (the agent) at house number three. There are only three homesteads on the market at the current time.

The home is a brick house, historic originating in 1893. A grand staircase wraps the foyer. A white front porch with massive pillars surrounds the front of the house, reminding me of the home in the movie, *Gone with the Wind*.

Family and friends believe a sensible house will serve me best given my current solo status. Yet, I am not limiting myself based on the square footage. Instead, I will ascertain what house is suitable.

Immediately, I feel an almost mystical atmosphere at this house.

The gardens bloom with colorful roses, dahlias, and giant blue hydrangeas.

A cornfield resides behind the house.

Tall pine trees surround the front of the property plus line the driveway.

The trees seem to whisper, "Welcome Home."

I feel like I am already home. Yet I tell Linda, "I need a sign, from above, to buy the house."

Within minutes, the rain begins. Soon, a heavy downpour occurs. Then, rapidly, a thick fog falls on the entire backyard. Now, Linda and I can barely see each other in the yard.

Although further away, the sky is crystal clear.

"I wish on a rainbow," I say to Linda.

I continue to repeat, "I wish *on a rainbow*."

After approximately ten minutes, a rainbow arrives. Then cascades across the front of the home and over the entire roof.

"I guess you got the rainbow," reacts Linda.

With a smile on my face, "I will take the house. Please submit an offer."

Sidebar – People have asked me how the Writer's Sanctuary originated. I found the premise of *Unexpected Miracles* to be at work. Because of this, I told God that I would use the house to heal myself and be a container for others to heal. Over the years, people arrived from various diverse locales, and many miracles occurred.

Reader Reflections, "Try to be a rainbow in somebody else's cloud." – Maya Angelou.

Chapter Eight

Planting New Seedlings

"The beautiful journey of today can begin
only when we let go of yesterday."
– Dr. Steve Maraboli

At times, my imagination gets the best of me. As a result, I tend to create scenes in my mind before they occur. I guess this attribute is a positive quality for a writer.

As I use my imagination, I transport myself to other periods—places where ancient rituals occurred, for example, Stonehenge and Edwardian times.

Nevertheless, I am confident that my current reality is in the present time.

On this specific morning, I don't feel myself. My abdomen is bloated, and I experience cramps in my uterus. Then while going to the bathroom, I realized that blood had arrived.

This experience can be a time of confusion for a young girl or a beautiful passageway into womanhood. In my

43

case, Mom hands me the book by Judy Blum, *Are You There God. It's Me Margaret,* a coming-of-age tale about puberty.

Our family does not typically talk about sexuality. Therefore, drafting an invite to a few of my closest friends to honor my first period is entirely out of the question!

After all, "I am raised with morals."

However, I decided to acknowledge this change in my life rather than ignore the gateway into womanhood.

The far back corner of our backyard is pretty private. Hence, a picture-perfect spot for performing a passageway ritual.

I locate a candle in the upstairs hall closet that Mom keeps there if an electric outage occurs. Collecting the candle, a journal, and pen, I walk to the backyard to start the ceremony.

I pluck a flower in route, but when I lay it on the ground, the flower appears to wilt.

A creek resides in the back area of the yard. I head there and select five stones.

Arranging the rocks in a circle, I place myself in the center.

I reach for my journal with an image of a dragonfly on the front and write the following, "*Dear God, are you there? It is me, Laura. You made me. Therefore, thank you. Honestly, I am not sure if this period will be significant pain. I want to recognize that I have the option to bear kids one day.*

However, not everyone is made for kids.

I want a dog, most likely—a lovely dog who can be my best companion.

For now, I hope I do not bleed through my shorts. PS, thanks for allowing me to blossom. We will see how I develop over time.

Shortly after, I realized that I was wearing white shorts and prayed that my menstrual time does not leak into a pair of shorts.

Even though it is daytime, I blow out the ceremonial candle. Afterward, I pick up the stones and return them to the creek but in a different formation.

I walk back to the house.

Mom inquires, "What are you doing?"

I reply, "I am planting seedlings."

For Reflection: "Keep planting, and sowing, living and knowing that beautiful things take time and that is okay." – Morgan Harper Nichols.

Later in life, I met Dr. Jill Little and Val Cook, who wrote an inspirational book, *Sharing the Medicine of Love*. I am their literary agent and publicist.

Dr. Jill and Val taught me the value of honoring rites of passage and creating sacred ceremonies.

During a gathering, they performed a ritual using a prayer shawl.

A woman in her sixties resides in a chair.

Val wraps the prayer shawl around the woman, covering the shoulders.

Sacred tobacco is lit. The space is blessed. Then all present (twelve women in total) share a ceremonial cup of tea.

To the woman clothed in the prayer shawl, Dr. Jill says, "Your lineage honors you. Now we celebrate the full essence of the beauty of who you are, where you have been, and what you are yet to experience in upcoming adventures."

Each attendee is encouraged to step forward and offer personal testimony, whether a shared memory or a positive character trait they have witnessed in the woman residing with the shawl.

This ceremony is hugely impactful, especially since my Mom is the woman residing in the circle. As a result, Mom experiences a deep sense of love and support.

Psychology Today communicates in *The Importance of a Ritual*, "One of the most important features of rituals is that they do not only mark time; they create time. By defining beginnings and ends to developmental or social phases, rituals structure our social worlds and how we understand time, relationships, and change."

Interesting Tidbit: "The Hopi Indians of Arizona believe that our daily rituals and prayers keep the world from slipping on its axis."

Points to Ponder: When was the last time you celebrated your journey? Or honored a rite of passage? A celebration could entail sitting with friends around a firepit to acknowledge the power of friendships.

Chapter Nine

The Kiva with Burning of the Ashes

"Do not heal the past by dwelling there; we heal the past by living fully present in the moment." – Marianne Williamson

An intuitive friend once said, "Connect with yourself at a deeper level. Go beyond the surface of your comfort zone. Release the past by bathing yourself in the newly found light."

Interpretation of literal comments is subjective. So, I chose to burn my sorrows away. Once the ashes burn, I can scatter the dust and rebirth myself.

Currently, I am in Tucson, Arizona. The desert cactus is in bloom; adobe-like casitas reside in the background. A walkable stone labyrinth is in the center courtyard, not far from my casita.

I walk the labyrinth (circular maze) intending to "Release the laden soot within me."

And to *"Find the light within."*

A journal is a nonjudgmental friend, so I scribe, "Why am I angry?"

Soon, I began to let go of the emotional baggage shoved deep inside of me. Stuff bottled up over time, ready to be set free.

At times, anger is not apparent; it can mask itself if stuffed in a box. One has to uncover the box's lid to allow breathing room to experience the emotion.

Also, anger can walk hand in hand with disappointment.

The feeling of disappointment is like crumbs of coffeecake, neatly brushed under the carpet. Until you pull back the rug and realize how much of a mess is there in the first place.

Then you obtain the vacuum and suck all the dirt into it. As a result, you are left with only remnants of dust. But instinctively recognize that emotions are more than specks on a clean white carpet from the shedding process.

Plus, a white rug never stays pristine.

Back to the current moment, I tear out five pages of journal writing that I have written and ignite the pages on fire. I do not encourage you to do this at home unless you have a container to hold the paper. I am sitting in front of a firepit, a kiva.

The fire pit is near the desert entrance that resides past the labyrinth, which I have been walking for three days.

I watch the journal pages burn, inch by inch.

Teardrops fall down the cheeks. I simply brush them off and return to observing the burning of my emotion.

I have burnt the anger out of me like a deep hallow. So consequently, light can finally shine into me.

Soon, the sky turns darkish in color.

Rain arrives to wash away the fragments of dirt that rise to the surface.

A complete cleansing occurs.

For Reflection: "We must be willing to get rid of the life we had planned to have the life waiting for us. The old skin has to be shed before the new one can come."
– Joseph Campbell

When you release that which no longer serves you, freedom arrives. You realize that the weight you have been carrying for far too long is gone. The burdens you once held have now dissipated.

Along the way, you understand that letting go and offering forgiveness frees you. Love holds the highest vibration transforming anger into forgiveness, disappointment into hope, and resentment into joy.

Inspired Idea: A simple affirmation statement is "**I am Love.**"

Chapter Ten

An Opportunity to Learn

"Every moment is a fresh new beginning." – T.S. Eliot

Before the Writer's Sanctuary, my boss's boss, I guess you could say top management called me in his office. He states, "We have the perfect assignment for you."

Instead of my risk aversion side spitting out "No," I arrive at John F. Kennedy Airport in New York City bound for London in the United Kingdom for a six-month work assignment.

Upon arrival at the London Heathrow Airport, a tall man wearing a worn wool hat holds up a sign marked with my surname, "Ponticello."

After collecting my luggage, we head towards the transport car. With an Irish brogue, he declares, "American? Here for work or pleasure?"

I answer, "Work."

The drive is silent.

Shaun, the driver, drops me off at the hotel. He pops open the trunk, grabs my suitcase, and bids me good wishes.

Immediately, I check into the hotel. Shower, and afterward, grab the piece of paper with the current work address that I had shoved into my purse.

I walk down four flights of stairs because the elevator appears broken. I start to sweat because my laptop case is too heavy from the corporate headquarters' loaner computer for this assignment.

After, I proceed to the white porcelain marble lobby, only to hail a cab to the new work location.

Immediately upon arrival, I noticed that not a single employee was dressed in colorful attire.

On the contrary, the typical dress code is monochromatic with gray slacks and a conservative white top. But I wore a fuchsia blouse and a pin-striped pantsuit with wedge heels.

I do not look the part of an Executive.

Instead, I appear more like a wet dog that needs a good shampoo. The rain on the way to work caused my wavy hair to frizz. Plus, the darn hair diffuser that took up too much space in the suitcase doesn't seem compatible with the electric outlet in the hotel bathroom.

Rachel from Human Resources greets me at the office. She offers me a cup of brisk British English with two sugar cubes.

I have always loved sugar cubes. As a young girl, I would sneak sugar cubes that resided in a silver bowl on the antique side buffet, at my Dad's aunt's house, into my pocket.

Back to today, I already have a sense of comfort at the London office with the sugar cubes and a brisk cup of English breakfast tea.

Until Rachel proclaims, "Never sit in front of a window in the city since the Irish Republican Army (known as IRA) is bombing random locations in London, as the conflict grows between Ireland and the United Kingdom, there have been recent bombings."

Before I can respond, my mind reverts to my Irish driver, who picked me up at the airport. He seemed sincere, yet, who knows.

I make a note of Rachel's comments.

Finally, I reply, "Okay. I got it."

I always request and sit at a table away from a window! (even today).

Work is intense due to long days.

During the weekends, I am alone for the first time in an exceptionally long time since the family has surrounded me in the past.

I walk in Hyde Park. Paved walkways, tall evergreen trees, and budding bushes line the park. On Saturdays, you might be lucky enough to observe the Queen's Mounties on horseback galloping during their return to Buckingham Palace.

I locate enchanting Art galleries.

For whatever reason, I experience great comfort in Art. When I sit on a bench in front of the art paintings, I swear that a voice emerges that murmurs how the image originates.

I eat modestly while in London. End up losing eight pounds since mad cow disease is rampant, and I am mostly consuming vegetables.

Once a week, I frequent a Chinese restaurant known for savory Peking duck with jasmine rice.

Walking distance from my lodging (known as a flat) is the most fabulous hotel in London, *The Dorchester,* that hosts afternoon tea. So, I head there and order a cup of Darjeeling tea.

Sitting in solace alongside a good book, *Pride and Prejudice* by Jane Austen, I envision myself sharing afternoon tea with the book's handsome leading character, Mr. Darcy.

Alternatively, the iconic rock singer, Rod Stewart, is in the sitting room at the Dorchester, where I am having tea.

You could not miss Rod. He has spiked blonde hair, tight jeans, a crisp white collar, a long shelve shirt, and wild-looking boots.

His strong personality appears to float across the sitting area.

I try to see if Rod is drinking tea in a porcelain cup. He probably prefers a stiff cocktail, such as a scotch on the rocks.

I tell the waitress, refiling my teacup, "I would like to meet Rod."

I realize that Rod is much better to spend time with than Mr. Darcy.

For Reflection: "I wish I knew what I know now before." – Rod Stewart

Points to Ponder: As you learn about yourself, what aspects of your life do you love? What areas could use a restart?

Chapter Eleven

Taking Chances

"In the end, we only regret the chances we didn't take." – Lewis Carroll

I've been reflecting on the concept of vulnerability. And the fact that any time change occurs, our psychological state undergoes a shift. That is why it is best to remember to *be kind to* yourself.

But to move forward, you have to take chances. For if you remain stationary, growth opportunities will pass you. You don't want to look back in life, saying, "I wish I had followed my intuition or taken a chance!"

I recall venturing outside my comfort zone. It was not an easy choice. It took courage to accept the work assignment in London, given numerous unknowns.

However, the experience provided me with an avenue to overcome fear and become comfortable with uncertainty.

Because life is an adventure, why not try something unfamiliar?

This attitude propelled me to The Louvre in Paris to meet the *Mona Lisa*.

I have to say that I was surprised by the scale of the artistic form.

I planted myself on a sitting bench near the *Mona Lisa* as if to sip a cordial together. Here, I stared deep into her eyes, and she appeared to recognize me for a minute. Yet, it was just the reflection of light in the room.

It might be helpful to explain how I arrived at the *Mona Lisa* in the first place. There was a fast-track train, a direct route from London to Paris. So, I bought a fare ticket. Before long, I departed the train station with the most decadent cup of hot chocolate in hand.

As soon as I arrived in Paris, I headed straight to the legendary gallery, Louvre Museum. I planned to meet the famous *Mona Lisa*, painted by Leonardo Da Vinci.

For me, she was the star of the show.

I thought she might remember me, but I recognized her. I had studied her years ago in an Art Literature class in College.

As a result, my obsession followed me all these years.

Interesting Tidbit: Considered an archetypal masterpiece of the Italian Renaissance, the Mona Lisa is "The best known, the most visited, the most written about, the most sung about, the most paradoxical work of art in the world."

Today, I sat gazing at her mystical smile as if a deep dark secret lured beneath the outer lining of her lips.

Art is subject to interpretation. She was chiseled just right. Constructed with flawless paint strokes, dripped in creation energy, and honed by the artist.

As I left the Museum, a notion arose that a picture is worth beyond a thousand words. And that a woman isn't defined by those who view her from afar. There is much more to a woman than her exterior veneer depicts. Her inner makings are the real masterpiece!

If Mona could speak in the present time, what advice does she offer?

Reader Reflection: "Wherever you go, go with all your heart." - Confucius

Point to Ponder: If presented the chance to follow your heart's desire, what would you do for a day?

Challenge for You: Visualize a dream of yours. Permit yourself to experience the feeling of joy as you leap into fields of possibilities that exist for you. Now take a small step to make that dream a reality. It could be as simple as cutting out an image of what represents your dream—or indulging in a conversation with a friend to share the goal.

Chapter Twelve

Discovery of Joy

"Discovering who you are today is the first step to being who you will want to be tomorrow." - Destiny's Odyssey

When I returned from my overseas assignment, I had to remind myself how to be. That comment probably seems ridiculous, but I spent a more significant amount of time than ever before with myself.

Assimilation back into the old never feels right. So, I began to explore, "What is next for me?"

I learned that I didn't want to get lost in work. It is essential to know that the work was intense. I averaged at least fifty-five to sixty hours of work a week to meet performance objectives. The stress took a toll. My health suffered.

Despite my earning income, I was willing to relinquish the security of a steady paycheck for freedom.

Life-altering decisions can shake us to the core. I leaped forward by leaning into my faith and unearthing self-belief. I quit a high-powered corporate job, started a business, and fell madly in love.

We married. Even in the face of our deep love, we divorced over time despite my resistance.

However, what I didn't comprehend at the time was that the most profound gift presented to me was an *opportunity for self-discovery.*

Through this journey, I found the rare pearl buried within me. It was hidden, stored deep within me until I dared to extract the beauty within.

This leads me to think of the Sea.

I first felt the mist of the Ocean when my parents took me to St. Petersburg Beach in Florida.

Dad was working in sales at the time and won a sales contest. While Dad attended work meetings, my sister and I built sandcastles on the shoreline outside our hotel and dove into waves. Mom sunned herself as she beamed with happiness.

Since that experience, I have always been fascinated by the Sea.

I am often standing at the water's edge, contemplating leaping into the depth of the waves.

Once fully engaged in the Sea, I search for signs of life, a shell hidden beneath the sand or a starfish.

I like the sound of a seashell as you place the shell up to the ear. Listening to the reverberation of the shell requires a person to be entirely still. Subsequently, you can hear the magic of the Sea's whisper.

Like the Ocean analogy, you reveal what lies under the surface of your being — realizing what feels magical for you.

You are permitting the tidal waves to wash away old debris.

You are welcoming the vitality of the Ocean's waves as a metaphor.

Each tidal wave delivers an ebb and flow pattern allowing you to release, heal, and invoke renewed energy.

Points to Ponder: If given a pearl, how would its qualities reflect you?

Could you notice the beauty within you?

What do you need to release into the Sea of Life?

Good Reflection: "Pearls don't lie on the seashore. If you want one, you must dive deep." – Chinese Proverb

Chapter Thirteen

Risks for Happiness

"What would life be if we had no courage
to attempt anything?"

– Vincent Van Gogh

Speaking of diving into the Sea, my
Mom's friend, Kathy, joins a travel group
after the loss of her husband.

She is hesitant at first, given that she
has only traveled with her husband in the
past. Finally, however, an opportunity
exists to step over fear and explore
different adventures.

Kathy develops confidence in meeting
friends. Shortly afterward, she goes on a
Viking Rhine River Cruise. Here she
meets Mary. They form a friendship
realizing that they have a lot in common.
Both are retired nurses, read fictional
books, and enjoy spending time with
their grandkids.

Before long, Kathy is renting a place in
Kissimmee, Florida, with Mary. All
because she took a risk!

Kathy shares, "I had to take a chance for joy. I could wither up after Clark's passing or obtain contentment in life."

She proceeds with a tear in her eyes, "Clark would want me to be happy. Each time I experience joy, I know my husband is smiling from above."

Why Taking Risks is Good for You states, "So why should you take risks in life? Enormous inner growth. It's in the uncertainty after a risk has been taken that personal growth is at its highest. We learn how to be content with our decisions, how to encourage ourselves to be optimistic about what the risk could contribute to the future, and how to adapt to big changes."

Melanie is another individual who took a risk. She joined one of my creativity workshops. Hence, I became familiar with her story.

Her sister, Sarah, was her best friend.

Although six years younger, later in life, they grew in friendship.

Their cousin owned a timeshare in Cabo San Lucas, Mexico. Therefore, they frequented. In the morning hours, with coffee in hand, they walked the sandy shores and discussed their dreams for the future. Then, as they watched the sunset, they laughed until their belly hurt from all the giggles and mint mojitos.

But unexpectedly, Sarah receives a cancer diagnosis.

Unfortunately, by this time, cancer had spread. And eventually, Sarah passes on.

Before passing, Sarah tells Melanie, "I will send a sign when I am gone. Accordingly, you will know that I am always with you."

After Sarah dies, Melanie is angry.

Melanie believes that she should have gone first, especially as the elder.

It takes Melanie four years to return to Cabo. Finally, having the courage to return there, Melanie walks the route she and her sister had traveled before now.

She encounters signs, a penny, and a flip flop that looks exactly like her sister wore. Almost immediately, the dolphin arrives. The dolphin is within three feet of the beach. The dolphin makes a motion to signal a wave with his fin.

Melanie knows these synchronicities are her sister sending signs. After this trip, she stops second-guessing everything.

"Anger festered too long in me after losing her. She would want me to take risks for happiness. I can't get back the past four years since her death, but I can find the joy in living life now," declares Melanie.

The great writer Anais Nan said, "And the day came when the risk to remain tight in a bud was more painful to remain in the bud."

Points to Ponder: There will always be instances where risk is required to move forward. If offered a chance to try something different, what would you do?

Chapter Fourteen

Writer's Circles, Friendships, and Confidence Building

"A single rose can be my garden... a single friend, my world." – Leo Buscaglia

By this time, life is moving forward. I am now leading creativity workshops at The Writer's Sanctuary.

I solicit Mom's help since she is available due to recent retirement. Also, Mom has the gift of hospitality. She loves to bake desserts and listen to stories; hence, she is a great job fit.

Plus, any opportunity to throw Jesus in the mix is a rare chance to bring another into God's good grace.

The authors adore Mom. She always goes the extra mile. For example, Mom memorizes their favorite drinks, pens name tags in calligraphy, and welcomes each participant with a smile.

I meet Thelma and Louise on this particular day, known as C and E. They are best friends, soul sisters, and co-authors of their book.

They arrive at class, pulling a black suitcase. It has pages & pages of their writings, and they both need to lift the bag into the house.

C says, "Hello. We are excited to be here. We brought all of our writings."

Let me set the scene that would take me a year to read. Multiple boxes of written materials, tape recordings, you name it, are located in their car plus in the suitcase that they wheeled into class.

I ring the angel bell that Mom gifted me, which signifies class to begin.

C writes down every single word that I utter. She is a teacher who takes outstanding notes.

She states, "I don't want to miss a word."

Mom passes brownies.

The authors break into subgroups.

They explore a writing prompt, which is simple, or so I believe. Next, I ask the class participants to describe their book on a single 5x7 index card. "Are we limited to one notecard? Could I possibly have five?" asks an author.

The writers encourage each other. Some of them cry in sharing their life stories. Now, Mom shares a box of Kleenex rather than brownies.

The male author who exposed his vulnerabilities during group discussion inquires, "Is there a social gathering after the class?"

Mom immediately responds, "Cheese and crackers, anyone? Beer and wine are in the kitchen."

Before communal time begins, the class participants assemble outside at the ancient rock circle.

Here, I have a crystal beacon. It is a copper structure with Lemurian crystals wrapped into a star of David symbol. Gathering stones, in particular six, surround the crystal beacon.

The authors place written intentions in a Tibetan bowl that resides in the center of the stones, below the crystal beacon.

Then, we collectively light intentions and hope the wind will carry our wishes out into the world.

I remind C and E that they cannot leave all their writings. Yet, I know from reading a few pages that there is a book in the making. This process starts a five-year journey that births a fantastic book that becomes a best seller.

I learn a lot from client work with C & E.

Friends can encourage each other even in the darkest of times. I witness their trust and respect for each other.

If you only in life have one person that believes in you, it can make a world of difference.

I remember like yesterday when C questioned her writing ability.

E imparts, "C, don't you understand?"

"No, what?" inquires C.

E continues, "You with a bag full of talents composed of all your gifts."

"I am getting forgetful in my old age," responds C.

E states, "Let me remind you. Laura, you tell her."

E adds, "A woman who knows her strength and compassion to love. Her courage to tell the story she must tell. I observe all of these facets in you."

C reacts, "Can you write this down?"

I start to laugh. At this point, after hours' worth of working, I could use a good glass of chardonnay.

This experience showcases the power of self-belief and the importance of a supportive cheerleading squad.

Can Happiness Lead to More Confidence? Yes, and Why informs, "The most important thing to remember about confidence is built by gaining experience and trust in your skills. By making a conscious decision to become happier, working towards your goal, and celebrating your successes, you are also building confidence."

Self Confidence Booster – Get in front of the mirror to affirm, "I am smart. I am happy. I am talented. I am worthy of incredible bliss."

Inspired Action: Who can you lean into for support?

Chapter Fifteen

Celebrate Everything

"It's a helluva start, being able to
recognize what makes you happy."
– Lucille Ball

Mornings are my thinking time. So, I like
to arrive at the office earlier than later.
When I first get to my office, I sit for a
few minutes and slowly drink my tea.
Then I review my calendar and formulate
a plan for the day.

Inside the top right drawer of my desk is
a bottle of lavender essential oil.

Lavender is known for its calming
properties. I inhale the scent when stress
arrives, which is frequent due to the
nature of the job.

A framed inspiration quote hangs on the
office wall from the anthropologist Jane
Goodall, who states, "Every single one of
us makes a difference on the planet
every day, and we choose the kind of
difference we make."

Today, my boss (in my corporate life)
named Jonathan asked to meet me.

I have a lot of respect for him. He is clean-cut, always sporting a long shelve shirt with silver cufflinks. Plus, dressed in gray slacks with shiny black loafers.

He drives a Volvo. My parking spot is three car lengths away from his spot in the lot, adjacent to our corporate office.

Management has its parking spots.

Given that both of us are punctual, I arrive outside his office at least fifteen minutes before the assigned meeting time.

He communicates, "Close the door."

I think, "Oh boy, this can't be good."

Usually, we always talk with the door wide open.

My boss conveys as he takes a sip of coffee, "I think it might be good to acknowledge the progress of the team and commemorate actions. What do you suggest?"

I request time to reflect on this question.

After, I head back to my office.

Sitting on my desk is a cactus plant since it requires little attention.

One of my staff members, John, shares, "At my last employer, there was a recognition system. When a staff member filled a job placement, everyone stood up and cheered."

John inspires me to acquire the cowbell.

I mount the bell outside my office door and call a staff meeting to share the recognition system.

Celebration of wins motivates staff plus brings people together.

When a staff member fills a job requirement compatible with the right candidate, they ring the cowbell. The team knows when the cowbell rings to stop what they are doing and start clapping. You can feel the excitement in the office when the cowbell rings.

The staff filled thirteen hundred jobs, given that the company expanded by leaps and bounds in the technical field. And each time, the cowbell rang.

Other leaders in the company learn about the recognition system. Then, almost immediately, they begin to install their reward system.

I mention this example because we tend to forget to celebrate accomplishments.

In *Three Reasons to Celebrate Little Victories,* "Progress on our goals makes us feel happier and more satisfied with life," writes Dr. Timothy A. Pychyl. "You don't have to wait for "someday" when you — hopefully — achieve your goal(s) to be happy. Instead, celebrate the small victories along the way and *be happy now.*"

Point to Ponder: Are you celebrating your growth? What if you sat for a few minutes and recognized progress by writing a thank you letter to yourself or the Universe?

Inspired Idea: Pen a Celebration Letter.

Dear Universe, I give gratitude for all the blessings in my life. Furthermore, I honor myself by stating that "I am an open vessel to receive more joy, prosperity, and well-being."

Chapter Sixteen

Barbie and the Power of Imagination

"The moment you doubt whether you can fly, you cease forever to be able to do it."- J. M. Barrie, *Peter Pan*

Even from a young age, I understood the power of imagination. I closed my eyes, visualized myself as a writer, and played out scenes.

Furthermore, my sister and I utilized our imagination during many playdates. Our beloved dolls, including Barbie, her best friend Mid, and Ken, the boyfriend, went everywhere with us.

We ventured to the backyard, the campfire at our friend's house, and the creek adjacent to our property for a dip in the stream. We hosted tea parties in our guest bedroom and danced together outside in Mom's garden.

Until the day arrived when Mom decided to host a garage sale, my imagination came to a dead halt.

"One person's discharge is another individual's fortune," says Mom about garage sales.

On this particular day, the weather is hot. As a result, there are zero airflows in the garage. And the plug-in fan that Mom insists will provide air circulation is making a terrible sound.

After two hours into the sale, an eight-year-old girl arrives with her Mom. They emerge from a station wagon.

The girl dresses in a plaid jumper.

Her Mom sports jeans with a T-shirt with an Aquarius sign on it.

The brother runs into the garage shouting, "Do you have any Barbie stuff?"

"Nope," I immediately respond.

The young girl reacts with a sad look, saying, "Oh, I want Barbie's dream house."

I thought to myself, "Oh no, not for sale."

Mom waves me over. "Laura, can you do me a favor and go upstairs to gather a few things to share with others," with a hand on her hip.

"For in giving to another, we give back to ourselves. That's Christ's way."

I can't stand when Mom throws Jesus in the mix.

Immediately, I know where this is going.

"You are getting a bit old for Barbie's dream house. It might be nice to help this young girl," invokes Mom.

"Are you kidding me?", as I storm upstairs.

My sister is at her friend's house currently. Instead, I am stuck helping Mom with the garage sale.

The next thing I know, the young girl's Mom states, "I have about thirteen dollars on me. Will you accept that amount?"

Before I could utter a word, the girl's brother packs up Barbie, Mid, Ken, and the dream house and loads them into their station wagon. They back out of the driveway waving goodbye.

I am devasted. Barbie and I voyaged around the world. I would constantly imagine the possibilities of where we could travel to in the future, such as the beach in Florida, London Bridge, Paris Eiffel Tower, anywhere, and one day we could go in our Camaro car and drive cross country.

My sister arrives home, and Mom shares, "Your sister decided to give Barbie and the Dream House to a family in need."

Christina's response is, "Can I get a pair of roller skates now?"

Obviously, not as devastated as I am.

Now, I have to create another way to use my imagination in exploration.

Books have become my passion.

I fell in love with *Nancy Drew and the Hardy Boys* series as if they were my best friends. While Barbie becomes a figment in my mind, I start to time travel with Nancy Drew as I read her stories. She is my type of gal – full of spunk!

As I grow into adulthood, I recognize the power of imagination, where stories can take you, and the ability to dream firsthand.

Points to Ponder: Where can your imagination lead you? If given a magic pen, what would you draw for yourself?

For Reflection: "With a bucket of Lego, you can tell any story. You can build an airplane or a dragon or a pirate ship; it's all whatever you can imagine." – Christopher Miller

Chapter Seventeen

Discovery Experiments

"Everything you could imagine is real."

– Pablo Picasso

I'm not sure what possessed me to study biochemistry in college. I wasn't terrific in science-related classes at the undergraduate level. Yet, I excelled in the arts, especially in English literature.

In hindsight, I probably should have chosen English as my major.

After the first semester, I knew biochemistry wasn't for me when I set the science lab on fire due to a mishap with the Bunsen burner.

Shortly after, my father received a bill for the accident. Consequently, it was time to select another major.

Later on, I understood that I had a spirit of curiosity—the desire to see how things evolved when mixed.

I suppose that is why currently, my garden is a playground to combine herbs and make tinctures since it's a living experiment.

When in the garden, I create unique formations. I study the sun patterns, talk to the plants, and become one with the flowers. Inspired ideas arrive like bursts of magic because of creative energy in the garden.

Remez Sasson shares in *The Power of Imagination and Mental Images* that "Imagination is a creative power that is necessary for inventing an instrument, designing a dress or a house, painting a picture or writing a book... What we often imagine and expect to happen can come into being."

Hence, I thought it might be fun to use our imagination as a propeller forward to explore the power of the mind to imagine.

Accordingly, we will be going on an imagination adventure. This endeavor can be done anywhere, in the office, at home, and outside in nature. Also, it might be nice to sit in a comfortable position and take a few deep breaths.

Discovery Imagination Exercise

Please Play-Along

First, let's start by relaxing. Let go of any tension in your body.

Know that the Universe is supporting you now, and all possibilities exist for you to create.

To help prepare for our adventure: silence all electronic devices.

To set the scene, the sky is crystal clear.

The sun is shining bright. A grass field is in front of you. And a giant oak tree is nearby, off in the distance.

You will use your imagination to move you forward as a burst of kinetic energy.

Here we go. You will tune in and tap into the power of imagination.

Action for You - Walk towards an oak tree (use your imagination to get there).

Imagine that underneath an oak tree is an effervescent bottle of golden liquid.

Reach for the effervescent golden liquid and spray it around you.

Since you have the power to create, a golden wheat field arises from beneath your feet when you spray the magical golden liquid.

The wheat appears to magnify in size and infuses a golden liquid into the air.

Allow your imagination to expand.

You begin to notice an exuberance forming.

Liquid gold is transmuting into liquid JOY.

You realize that you are absorbing JOY.

You are ingesting into your essence, cellular memory, and into your aurora the feeling of Joy. You experience a conscious energy expansion, and the golden wheat field seems infinite in scale.

You realize that being JOYFUL is a beautiful feeling.

Let yourself experience exuberance.

Your powers are limitless. You can paint, draw, dance, fly or walk around in this creative landscape of Joy.

When ready, shift your attention back to the Oak Tree, where we first began. Don't worry. Your imagination will transport you to the branches and the strength of the tree's trunk.

Action for You – Envision yourself sitting under the Oak Tree. Notice the solid supportive trunk of the tree. Its branches offer you shelter and induce a spirit of tranquility. Vibrancy surrounds you; the grass is green, and flowers sprout in iridescent blue, red, and pink colors. At this moment, you feel the support of Mother Earth, and creative sparks begin to formulate.

Take a few breathes.

When ready, return to the current time reality. Anchor your feet on the ground and tap your feet. Open your eyes if closed. Become mindful of your present surroundings. For example, look around the room or the environment you reside in now.

Challenge for You – Given what you just experienced, you may want to include more "imagining" into your everyday life, if even for a few minutes. Remember, imagination can take us to wonderful discoveries.

Also, you can return to this exploration exercise to play and create.

The key in this imagination exercise is to get you out of the brain's logical thinking part and encourage you to tap into the playful arena of creativity that exists in all of us.

Additionally, you can spray liquid joy onto your essence whenever you need a burst of JOY.

Inspired Idea: If you need a boost of playfulness, activities with kids are super fun. Create art, build sandcastles, make cookies, or just observe the power of laughter. And oh – watch a movie; the animation world is a wonderful way to transport the imagination.

Chapter Eighteen

Lakeside Vistas

"What would it be like if I could accept life – accept this moment - exactly as it is?" – Tara Brach

I needed a pause from the world around me. Therefore, I drove to the Lake, which was not far from my house. As soon as I stepped out of the car, the sunshine welcomed me. That's when I noticed the brilliance of the Lake glistening in front of me.

In the distance, yet close enough to see, is a border collie dog wagging its' tail.

An older gentleman sits on a park bench reading the *New York Times.*

A perfect day exists for an artist like Norman Rockwell. If Norman were alive, he would construct a masterpiece of art from this scenery.

A young girl in a bright pink t-shirt with black leggings is flying a kite. The multicolored kite that she holds begins to soar when a gust of wind arrives from the Lake's eastern shore.

Meantime, boats in the background are zipping along the shoreline.

The girl with the kite picks up her pace and begins to run. Finally, her mother calls out, "Run faster."

The girl heads towards the boat dock and looks directly at me with a smile.

After a few minutes, she stops abruptly.

Her kite begins to drop lower until it eventually falls on the green grass in the park.

Her mother inquires perplexingly, "Why did you stop running?"

"Momma, you run from place to place. I noticed the wrinkles of stress on your face. I like our life best when things are less hectic. As I ran, I thought, What if I stop what I am doing, sit still, and become aware of what happens," says the girl.

She continues, "I have to tell you that it is pretty awesome to reside here with my legs crossed. I can hear the whispers within me telling me to slow down. I even noticed the seagulls in the sky."

For Reader Reflection – What if you pause long enough to notice the world around you?

As I returned to my car, I couldn't stop thinking about the sage advice offered by this girl.

Soon my thoughts shifted to a memory of a friend and former colleague, Susan.

Susan is a single mom, and her son is the love of her life. She is full of energy and makes me laugh.

She shows up with bite-sized treats of Ben & Jerry's Cherry Garcia® Ice Cream when work is stressful to help brighten our day. Now for a lactose intolerant person, the consumption of ice cream is not the smartest choice. Unfortunately, frozen yogurt options are not readily available. But I indulge anyways.

Susan always offers me the first bit of ice cream. She never helps herself. Instead, Susan waits for me to start eating before helping herself.

Finally, after doing the same a third time, I say, "Help yourself first."

"No, you go ahead," Susan replies.

We repeat this cycle multiple times.

My Mom is similar to this type of woman who is constantly feeding the needs of others before her own. However, there is a delicate balance between helping another and taking care of yourself.

For Reflection: "Bottom line, don't expect to drink from an empty cup!"

Points to Ponder: If you don't care for yourself, who will? What self-care practices can you incorporate into your daily routine?

Chapter Nineteen

Gratitude

"When I started counting my blessings,
my whole life turned around."

– Willie Nelson

I remember planting a hundred zinnia seeds. Finally, a patch of land was perfect for growing the flowers. So, I spread the soil, covered the seedlings with dirt, and asked the Universe to make them grow.

However, I didn't expect the weeds to overtake the garden. I began to obsess about the weeds instead of appreciating the beauty of the flowers. So, I lost perspective.

This analogy reminds me of Jim. He runs a successful business in town, has a fierce dedication to his family, and knows when to care for himself.

The golden rule to happiness is to "Give gratitude," Jim offers.

"By six am in the morning, I have a cup of coffee in hand. The kids are still sleeping. Consequently, I have time to reflect. The first thing I do is to say Thank you, God, for this life."

"On days when I struggle, I think of one thing to acknowledge from a perspective of gratitude."

After all, *"Gratitude is attitude!"*

Before we part ways, Jim imparts, "Find the bright light in a day. **Thank your lucky stars that you have a brand-new start today."**

Robert Emmons, a leading gratitude researcher, has conducted multiple studies on the link between gratitude and well-being. His research confirms that gratitude effectively increases happiness and reduces depression.

For Reflection: "How you treat yourself is how you are inviting the world to treat you." – Unknown.

Point to Ponder: What gratitude practice can you begin?

Chapter Twenty

Random Acts of Kindness and Notes of Thanks

"There are those who give with joy, and that joy is their reward." - Khalil Gibran

My friend Myron volunteers his time to drive the bus for *Meals on Wheels*. He is an electrician with tons of work commitments. However, he sets aside time to help others.

One day, his friend Jack states to Myron, "Why you do it – give all your time? Don't you just want to hunt or go fishing? I barely have time for myself."

Myron reacts, "When I help another in need, it makes me happy. I see them struggling to get out the door and into the van. And I know that that will be me one day, and I will need a helping hand."

Action for Happiness reveals in *Why Helping Others Matter*, "Helping others is good for them and a good thing to do, but it also makes us happier and healthier. Giving also connects us to others, creating stronger communities and helping to build a happier society for everyone. ... So, if you want to feel good, do good!"

Reading is another act of love. As you sit with a sick friend or a grandchild, you experience a human connection.

Empathic words go a long way. A simple gesture towards another can brighten their day and lend a helping hand.

Let's assume there are days when we can use a little cheering up, whether a phone call from a friend or a random stranger holding the door at the grocery store. These acts of kindness mean a lot.

"For in giving to another, we receive much more than we expected."

I learned this lesson early on from Mom.

While in my younger years, I wished that I was roller-skating with the other kids in the neighborhood instead of volunteering with Mom at the church bake sale. After hours of baking cookies in preparation for the bake sale, it brought Mom great satisfaction when her last cookie sold.

She always had a massive smile in the car on our ride back home.

Soon to follow, I knocked on doors with Girl Scout cookies in hand to raise funds for our local troop. Meantime Dad pedaled chocolate mint cookies at work to help my efforts, and Mom cheered me on to achieve the fundraising goal.

Then the moment arrived when I had only one box of cookies left to sell.

Penny was an older woman in the neighborhood. All I honestly wanted to do was unload the last box of cookies. I was tired and ready to head back home. But Penny insisted that I come inside for a cup of hot chocolate.

As she stirred the marshmallows in the steaming hot cup, she said, "It's good of you to visit me. Ever since my Chuck passed away and my daughter moved, I have felt lonely."

As I waited for the hot chocolate to cool, I noticed her book collection. One of my favorite books was on the bookshelf, *Little Women* by Louisa May Alcott.

Penny begins reading an excerpt to me after I mention my affection for the story. The passage states, "Oh, Jo. Jo, you have so many extraordinary gifts; how can you expect to lead an ordinary life? You're ready to go out and find a good use for your talent. Tho' I don't know what I shall do without my Jo. Go, and embrace your liberty. And see what wonderful things come of it." – Louisa May Alcott, *Little Women.*

Little does Penny realize; that Jo is one of my favorite characters in the book. I like Jo's character because she dares to take a risk and wants to become a writer.

After listening to Penny read, I make room in my bike basket for the copy of *Little Women* that Penny bestows on me.

And also, the money for the sale of the last box of cookies. What a triumphant day!

Point to Ponder: What random act of kindness could you perform? Simple gestures mean a lot to people.

A Note of Thanks

"The joy we feel has little to do with the circumstances of our lives and everything to do with the focus of our lives."
— Russel M. Nelson

I love to receive cards scribbled with notes. The sheer fact that a friend or reader took the time to write an inscription is like providing me with a pot of gold.

I once supported an executive who consistently made writing thank you notes. For example, he penned a card to employees who positively impacted customers.

His putting pen to paper meant a lot to the receivers. In addition, his signature on the note with a few words shows leadership commitment.

"When I receive a token of gratitude, in the form of a thank you card, it makes me feel like the company values me," said Jared.

In a world that entails texting, instant messaging, and multiple social media platforms, mechanisms do exist for you to share thanks in the form of a few lines.

Yet, there is energy in a handwritten note.

Psychology Today in *Handwritten Notes Have Surprising Consequences* imparts, "Researchers found that prosocial gesture of expressing gratitude in a handwritten note boosts positive emotions and well-being for both the letter-writing expresser and the recipient of stated appreciation."

Point to Ponder: When was the last time you communicated with a loved one, friend, or staff member? And shared how they matter to you?

Chapter Twenty-One
A Brand-New Canvas

"Every canvas is a journey of its own."

– Helen Frankenthaler

Experiences provide a backdrop for life. But history does not define you! Instead, you can create what makes sense for you. The current moment presents an opportunity to experience life from a new pair of looking glasses.

Therefore, I am going to hand you a blank canvas.

You don't need to be a master artist.

Instead, start simple with one aspect of life you desire to draw. Maybe it's a secret longing you have stored inside you, ready to come to fruition. Or an element of daily living that you want to incorporate.

To explore this concept, I sat down with a client, Suzanne, and asked, "What would you paint into your life when presented with a blank canvas?"

Immediately she answered, "A renovated kitchen. Since the kitchen represents the gathering space for our family, I would love an updated kitchen island that encourages us to cook food and share experiences."

Shortly following, Suzanne found a piece of art at a local consignment store with an image of Tuscany.

During our conversation, Suzanne noted that she wanted to incorporate other brushstrokes into her life.

Suzanne has always wanted to study international cooking. The art image on the kitchen wall now serves as a visual for a future goal to attain, to attend cooking school in Italy.

While not everyone is jumping on a plane to find their nirvana, this example demonstrates the power to create your brand-new canvas—one idea at a time.

This leads me to Julie. Julie was an investment banker and loved to craft pretty much anything. So, she made friends and family sweaters and blankets; she called them Cozy Cots.

Because wrapped in her blanket, you felt cozy, even if you were on a cot.

When I discussed the idea of the brushstrokes of her life, she said one word, "Unfinished." Then she drew a circle.

Julie told me, "Life is fluid. My past does not define me or even the choices I have already made. Instead, I have the chance to *rebirth each day*."

She continues, "Today, I will paint a sunset with two little umbrellas inside a wine glass. One umbrella will signify relaxation since I work too much, and the other will represent the unknown of what is left to drink in the game of life."

Points to Ponder: How will you construct the painting of your life? What colors can you paint into your life?

"Life is not a journey to the groove with the intention of arriving safely, in a pretty and well-preserved body. But rather to skid in broadside, thoroughly used up, totally worn out, and proclaiming, "Wow, what a ride." – Robert Fulghum

Chapter Twenty-Two

The Blue Bird

"I wake up every day and think, "I'm breathing. It's a good day." – Eve Ensler

Nana Rose always encouraged me to be the best version of myself. My family believes that I inherited Nana's hazel eyes, but instead, I received her tenacity, although my eyes are hazel.

As I reflect on memories of Nana, a smile encompasses my face.

Nana was a fantastic baker. A fan favorite is sugar cookies in the shape of an S with green sprinkled sugar. Plus, anise cookies, according to Mom, are ideal for dipping in tea first thing in the morning. So, all I know is I grew up eating succulent baked goods.

When she mixed cookie creations, Nana sang out the kitchen window.

She had the voice of an angel. Almost immediately, the blue jays would hear Nana's voice and start to arrive. At one point, I counted close to six blue jays outside the kitchen window.

Nana was married to Papa John, the family's bread earner. He was a foreman at the local optical factory. He worked a second job selling real estate for extra money since Papa John is particularly good at connecting with people.

When my sister and I stayed over for sleepovers, Papa arranged the rabbit antenna ear affixed to the top of their family television. We would gather, and dance as music blared from The Lawrence Welk Show and Star Search, both music variety talent shows.

Papa was an exceptional dancer.

"Twinkle Toes," the family called him.

He taught my sister and me the Cha-Cha-Cha dance. In a rhythmic movement, one step ahead, two steps back, three steps forward.

Nana has lots of curves in her body. At first, she did everything in her might to shake her hips. Once she moved, she pivoted back and forth like a spinning top as the music played. We danced in delight.

I felt a tremendous amount of love between Nana and Papa. They would hug each other and share why they felt blessed to be part of the family.

Like every family, there is no perfect storm. Nana received a Breast Cancer diagnosis. However, she does not feel sorry for herself.

She acquired strength from her faith.

"God willing, I will celebrate each day" is her mindset.

The most specific childhood memory is Nana nurturing her three-rose garden on the right side of their ranch house. All the roses are pink in color.

"To care for a garden is to tend to the soul," Nana said.

Nana grabbed my hand when the rain fell and took me to the side rose garden.

With conviction, she conveyed words that still ring true, "Without the rain, the flowers won't grow. There will be challenging times in life but remember your strength."

"The rain serves a purpose in life. When the rain passes, the sun will emerge. Plus, the rain nourishes the flowers to grow," said Nana.

As I look back at these special times with Nana and Papa, I recognize that they did not have a lot of materialist items.

Instead, they had simple occurrences with **joy** that fed them.

They are not afraid to get stains on the light-colored carpet.

Or welcome in strangers in need.

They look at life as though the glass is half full instead of half empty. And fortunately, this mindset always gets them past the hard times.

As time goes on, Nana dies.

I took the news extremely hard, as I was twelve years old.

Mom told me, "Her spirit will live on."

Frankly, I did not believe Mom.

The funeral home was depressing. I hate to say it. I refused to witness her lying in the black coffin.

Mounds of floral arrangements lined the interior entrance and surrounded Nana's coffin.

You would think a queen passed.

Instead, she was an ordinary woman who did extraordinary things because she offered encouragement when speaking with people.

Years later, I found myself at a local retreat center not too far from my house.

On this particular day, the blue sky is pristine. The vista is breathtaking. In the background is Skaneateles Lake with its crystal-clear waves of water.

A white gazebo adorns the property and sits adjacent to the lake water.

I decide to walk toward the pavilion.

Five blue jays fly near me. No matter which direction I walk, blue jays appear.

They are pursuing me at one point.

I swear I hear my Nana's voice when the blue jays make their chirping noises.

At this point, only a single bird remains; the other four have flown away.

The blue jay comes within inches of my shoulder as if to give me a hug of support.

I sense Nana's presence, and I know she is sending me a sign from above.

Nana is fluttering her wings near me.

Something in me changed that day. I attained hope in the bustling of nature.

For Reflection: "A bird sitting on a tree is not afraid of the branch breaking, because her trust in not in the branch, but in her own wings."- Unknown

Tidbit: In Celtic symbolism, the blue jay is believed to carry messages between dimensions. Blue Jays are also considered guardians and helpers of people on spiritual journeys.

Chapter Twenty-Three
Bursts of Joy

"Joy blooms where minds and hearts are open."- Jonathan Lockwood Huie

With creative energy, anything in life is possible. Hence why, I favor my star-powered floral t-shirt. Let me tell you, I feel invincible when I wear it. Rainbow colors weave into the soft fabric.

On the back of the shirt is a saying, "Grow Seeds of Hope."

After working hard in the garden, I reward myself with black raspberry ice cream. But, because Bunny is a good girl, she does not get the chocolate cone—in its place, a vanilla ice cream with a doggie treat.

On days when the rain falls, I retreat inward. In the silence, I can hear the beating of my own heart and the musings within me.

A journal has always been a friend because it does not judge. In *Five Powerful Health Benefits of Journaling,* "What's more, journaling unlocks and engages right-brained creativity, which gives you access to your full brainpower. Truly, journaling fosters growth."

Flowers on my desk serve as a mood lifter. It is amazing how uplifting a single bud can be.

A sticker of a gal sitting in meditation resides on my computer. This visual reminds me to take time for self-care practices.

In addition, I have a joy water bottle. On the front of the bottle is an image of a sunflower.

Each time I drink from the cup, I see myself ingesting JOY. Plus, water is a good energy source for the body.

Points to Ponder: What else can you place into a cup of JOY that are daily practices providing you a chance to experience life from a perspective of joy?

Inspired Idea - What about creating a joy water bottle for yourself? And each time you ingest the water, you feel a splash of joy.

Chapter Twenty-Four

Sustaining Tools for Daily Living

"Happiness is an inside job. Don't give anyone else that much power over you."
– BestofLife.com

Even though I adore sparklers, I recognize that life isn't always full of sugar plum fairies and sparklers that light up the night sky.

Challenges can arise. However, you have learned that bits of joy help you weather the heavy showers in life.

Because it's easy to forget and helpful to remember, I thought it might be beneficial to offer a few reminders.

First, you did a fantastic job at facing adversity in life. Did you hear me? You did a remarkable job at becoming the person you are now!

While all life lessons create who you are, a fresh beginning exists at the onset of each day. Thus, start your day with positivity.

Given life is worth living, crank up the music and be the maestro of your life.

Walk barefoot in the green grass.

Taste the saltness of the Sea's air.

Ride the wave of the rollercoaster.

Try various occurrences even if you are afraid.

Project Happiness reveals, "The only way you will ever notice opportunities arise is if you are willing to look at life as a river with boats full of chances passing you by. You need to be the one to jump from the shore straight onto those opportunity boats because if you hesitate, you'll miss out on what could be a life changer!"

Even if yesterday was not the best day, *today is a restart* - a chance to embrace life from a space of joy.

Choosing joy is not selfish. As a matter of fact, the exact opposite. When you evoke joy, you offer the world a gift. Moreover, since joy is transformative, those around you will also experience your happiness.

Here is to YOU... a toast to honor the fullness of your essence.

For life stands still, and a river of love flows from the world to you and from you to the world.

Inspired Idea: Celebrate YOU! Do something just for you that makes you feel joyful.

"Our path to reach out to the stars should be full of celebrations, the journey is the most beautiful part of these dreams." – Purvi Raniga

Afterward – What's Next?

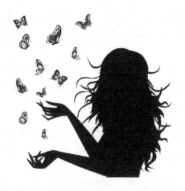

"Today is the first day of the rest of your life." – American Proverb

Writers like to edit their work forever; hence, I am not an exception. But instead of getting caught up in the overedit process, I would like to focus on the book's original purpose: to help you create a pathway to JOY.

As you become aware that you are worthy of joy, you start to live from a space of blissfulness.

You say "No thank you" to the stuff you once said Yes to, and you muster the courage to take time for yourself.

You discover opportunities to experience life from a fresh perspective. For example, you notice the sparrow's nest on your front porch, the flowering tree on the street, and the other aspects of life that you may have overlooked.

Furthermore, you become aware of the small pleasurable aspects of life. For example, a hug from your child, a walk with your dog, or sitting with a cup of coffee in hand can create delight.

As you venture forward, remember to leap into fields of self-discovery.

The best friend you will ever have is yourself. So why not spend time together?

You will discover that a deep well of knowledge exists within you, and innate longings are ready to emerge if you listen.

Take a chance for joy. You have this life; therefore, make the most of it.

As my dear friend Barbara says, "Paint unicorns all over the walls of the sky. Travel to places within yourself where magical wonderlands exist as if you are discovering life for the first time."

♥ ♥ ♥

Recently, I decided to commemorate the completion of this book because it's good to celebrate.

As I finished the book's last line, I took a few moments to reflect. Writers are an interesting bunch. We pour ourselves inch by inch into the canvas of our stories, feel incredibly vulnerable, shed pages of work, then arrive at the understanding that we've done the best we can do for now.

And along the way, we transform.

For, I am not even the same person who started this book. I have a few more strands of gray in my hair that I tend to masquerade with color. Additionally, I have shifted from wearing tighter clothes to selecting more flowy attire that somehow induces my creative mojo.

Through self-reflection, I acknowledge that I am but a kite that starts slowly blowing in the wind until she gathers enough momentum to soar to new heights. So, I breathe in life with the wind at my back – only to savor the exact moment when life breathes into me.

Then there is a conversation, a self-monologue, surrounding the evolution of my younger self with my wiser imperfect self. Both forms are etched into me, and I realize that somehow, the intersection of the fullness of who I am – is still evolving.

My mind recalls that today is a chance to honor the writer's journey. Therefore, I have decided to hold a festive party.

I invite a most distinguished guest to the party, my faithful companion, Bunny. Her party dress entails a purple sparkle dog collar and her natural look; after all, the Vizslas have green eyes and rust-colored hair. She doesn't necessarily need to put on any makeup.

Alternatively, I selected a comfortable pair of yoga pants with a kaleidoscope of color. And a black tunic top feels perfect for this occasion.

I pull my hair back and insert the turquoise hairpin that I kept hidden in a jewelry box. It is symbolic, given that it's an heirloom gift from my mother. And I put on length extending mascara, which is like icing on a cake, the finishing touch.

In preparation for the festivities, before this moment, I walked down the hall, unfastened the China cabinet door, and selected two plate settings (one for me and one for Bunny).

Both plates have a rose floral pattern.

The rose pattern signifies the flower within me waiting to blossom. Plus, I inherited China from Nana Rose.

I place an Irish linen tablecloth on the kitchen mahogany table, acquired during my time in London. In the center of the table, I set a vase of fresh sunflowers since flowers make me happy. Yesterday, a local farmer happened to place them roadside around the corner from my homestead.

Then, I selected a few pieces of decadent Godiva® chocolate recently sent to me by my publishing attorney. I love chocolate, especially the truffle kind that, with each bite, a magic surprise awaits you. But, since I didn't want Bunny to feel left out, I put salmon treats on her plate instead of chocolate.

Music begins to play to set the mood. In particular, a song by Stevie Nicks, *Edge of Seventeen.* Immediately, Bunny starts to nod her head as if the music inspires her. Soon, we both begin to groove to the beat. Bunny is tapping her paw, and me, my feet.

I lift a crystal wine glass and sip chilled Riesling while savoring every drop.

Simultaneously, Bunny licks her lips with pure delight from the salmon treats.

Shortly following, Bunny smiles at me.

She knows me best. In these moments, Bunny imparts, "What a road we traveled to arrive here now. We questioned many times where the path was leading us. Tired, wet, and full of optimism, we mustered the courage to keep on trucking through the rain in hopes of the rainbow. And we finally found that joy was awaiting our arrival."

After all, when you spend this much time together, you get to know each other's sentiments.

Plus, dogs have a particular language that their owners understand well.

After sharing her insight, Bunny signifies that she wants to be excused from the table. I can tell she has to use the bathroom. So, I open the patio door adjacent to the kitchen, and Bunny runs out.

Taking her sweet time, I step outside only to find that Bunny resides in the garden of happiness. Just months before, I had planted seedlings. Today, of all days, the butterfly is fluttering its wings on a newly formed blossom.

For Reflection: You are but the butterfly. Constantly changing form and becoming that which you are destined to be. So don't be afraid, for your wings have already formed. But, if for a moment, you forget, look for a sign, and I shall be there to remind you of your iridescent splendor.

Addendum – Refreshments for Joyful Living

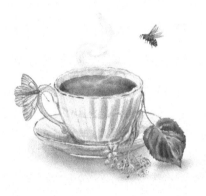

"Pull up a chair. Take a taste. Come join us. Life is endlessly delicious."

– Ruth Reichl

Refreshments along with bite-sized finger sandwiches are pleasant at gatherings.

Accordingly, it might be nice to provide some nourishment, as well.

You and I first began our journey with a bit of excitement. I invited you to sip the content of this book. Also, to absorb what felt right to you as you navigated forward.

By now, you know, "When you take time to replenish your spirit, it allows you to serve others from the overflow. You cannot serve from an empty vessel." - Eleanor Brown.

In doing so, you commit to hydrating.

Afterward, you can water those around you. As you refresh, you find chances for self-nourishment. Be willing to carve out time, no matter what, for you.

Make sure to rejuvenate when you need a bit of encouragement.

Water the garden of your heart.

Drink from life's intoxicating instances.

Inhale the fragrances of the blessings arising from your daily occurrences.

Look for the gift at this moment.

And know that your cup of joy is always overflowing.

Help Spread Joy

"Joy is not in things; it's in us."

- Robert Wagner

I could use your help since the world can experience more JOY. Therefore...

If inspired, please tell a friend about your experience with this book.

To help spread the word, purchase *The Book of Joy, Overcoming Life's Obstacles* as a gift for friends, family, colleagues, and staff, or donate to a local library.

Reviews do help. Post a book review on Amazon.com and share it on social media pages.

I want to hear about your experiences.

So please invite me to your book club, event, organization, or business since we can uplift each other collectively.

Most importantly, let's be sparks of light for the world to see that joy is possible.

With gratitude to you, XO, Laura

Book Sources/Endnotes

Kelly Bilodeau, Harvard Women's Health Watch,https://www.health.harvard.edu/b log/want-more-happiness-try-this-202107022522

How Being Present Will Bring Joy to Your Life, medium.com/mindcafe/how-being-present-will-bring-joy-to-your-life-c0f80ca8d80b

Serena Williams and The Art of Visualization,https://thedailycoach.subst ack.com/p/serena-williams-and-the-art-of-visualization#

5 Reasons to Take a Breath Before Responding,theleaderslocker.com/2011/ 08/22/5-reasons-to-take-a-breath-before-responding

The Importance of a Ritual www.psychologytoday.com/us/blog/anth ropology-in-mind/202005/the-importance-ritual

Mona Lisa, wikipedia.org/wiki/Mona_Lisa

Why Taking Risks is Good for You, https://shop.projecthappiness.org/blogs/

project-happiness/why-taking-risks-is-good-for-you

Can Happiness Lead to More Confidence,www.trackinghappiness.com/can happiness-lead-to-confidence

Three Reasons to Celebrate Little Victories,www.shawnellis.com/celebrate-little-victories

Power of Imagination www.successconsciousness.com/blog/concentration-mind-power/power-of-imagination

7 Incredible Benefits of Gratitude, https://doctorHealsMind.com/7 incredible-benefits-of- gratitude

Why Helping Others Matters, www.actionforhappiness.org/10-keys-to-happier-living/do-things-for-others

Handwritten Thank-You Notes Have Surprisingly Positive Consequences, www.psychologytoday.com/us/blog/the-athletes-way/201808/handwritten-thank-you-notes-have-surprising-consequences

Bird Guide, thebirdguide.com/blue-jays-symbolism

Five Positive Health Benefits of Journaling,https://intermountainhealthca re.org/blogs/topics/live-well/2018/07/5-powerful-health-benefits-of-journaling

Acknowledgments

"A community is like a ship; everyone ought to be prepared to take the helm."
– Henrik Ibsen

In creating this book, I am grateful to many people:

Mom and Dad for years of self-sacrifice to provide the best life for their daughters.

To my cherished sister, Christina, thank you for being an unwavering support cheerleader in my life.

Nana Rose and Papa showcased that laughter is a Band-Aid for all wounds and taught me to embrace simple pleasures.

Bunny - Oh, the places we have gone and the adventures yet to arrive. You are an angel in my life.

Sheila Applegate, dear friend, founder of Consciously Awesome®, and my creativity coach thank you for helping awaken my sleeping Creative Muse. I am forever grateful to you.

John Sammut, my financial planner, thank you for gifting me "*The War of Art, Breaking through Blocks and Winning*

Your Creative Battles" by Steven Pressfield. This book is about overcoming resistance and inspired me.

Christopher Moebs for his talents in creative cover design and production.

And to all the amazing artists who contributed to the images in this book.

Becky (Rebecca) Orsi, a great teacher, suggested the title for the Five-Minute Positivity Pause; thank you.

Thank you, John, Traci, Chris, and Elizabeth, my clients who mean the world to me. Together we encourage each other. And there are more stories to tell.

I am grateful to the authors/speakers who took the time to provide endorsements. You inspire me with your stories.

About Author

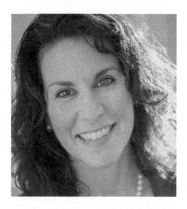

Laura is a coach, award-winning and bestselling author, lecturer, and teacher who resides in Owasco, New York, with her Vizsla dog, Bunny. Together they experience adventures while chasing butterflies and walking in nature.

Her journal is still a beloved friend, and she rejoices in creating beauty in the garden.

Laura's upcoming book will be *The Road Back Home,* about her story of discovering herself again and the true meaning of life.

Given that each of us has the wisdom to share, Laura looks forward to learning about your joyful story. Connect on social media and **lauraponticello.com**